CANADIAN ENGLISH LANGUAGE BENCHMARK ASSESSMENT FOR NURSES (CELBAN)

PREPARATION GUIDE

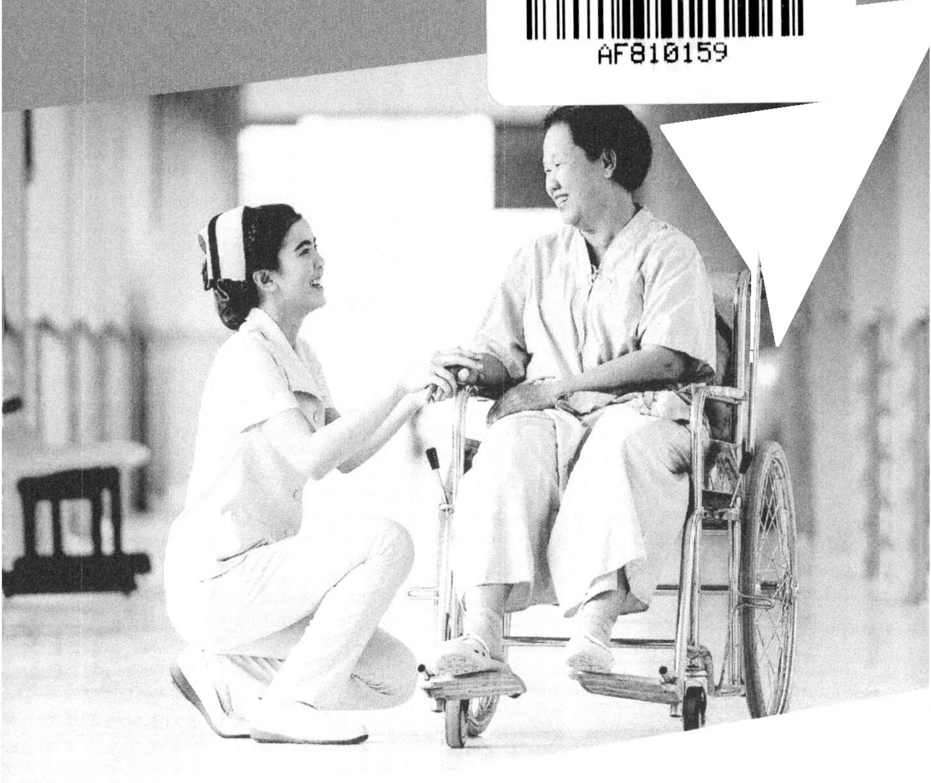

Marilyn McGreer

Canadian English Language Benchmark Assessment for Nurses (CELBAN)
Preparation Guide

Published by Marilyn McGreer, St. Albert, Canada.

ISBN 978-1-9994788-3-4

Publication assistance by
PAGEMASTER PUBLISHING
PageMasterPublishing.ca

ABOUT THE AUTHOR

Marilyn McGreer is a home economist and educator in the fields of early childhood and nursing. She began her nursing career in 2003 as a graduate from the Practical Nurse Program at NorQuest College, Edmonton, Alberta, and obtained nursing specialty in immunization and foot care nursing. Upon graduation she worked as a Licensed Practical Nurse in both acute care and long-term care facilitates.

Marilyn has a Bachelor of Science degree in Home Economics, with specialization Family Studies, from the University of Alberta. In addition to nursing, she worked as an educator and supervisor of children and adult learners in a variety of settings, including daycare centers and post-secondary institutions. She holds the designation Professional Home Economist and level three certification as an Early Childhood Educator.

For the past ten years, she has enjoyed working as a career coach, mentoring and teaching English to internationally educated nurses preparing to write CELBAN. She is the president of the Vocational Pathways Association of Edmonton.

ABOUT VPAE

Vocational Pathways Association of Edmonton (VPAE) was formed to support and assist new Canadians in removing barriers to employment in Canada, focusing on internationally educated nurses.

Training is available through VPAE to prepare internationally educated nurses to pass CELBAN and to assist them in improving the use of their English language skills in their daily lives.

One ways to prepare for the exam is to take the practice exam (the Institutional CELBAN). The practice exam uses the same format as the official exam and is the best tool to assess your readiness for the official exam.

To register for either the practice exam or a two-hour tutoring session, visit the VPAE website at www.vocationalpathways.ca or contact Marilyn at 780-920-5335.

VPAE is located at 13535 - 122 Avenue, Edmonton, Alberta.

CONTENTS

CHAPTER ONE
INTRODUCTION

The *Canadian English Language Benchmark Assessment for Nurses (CELBAN) Practice Guide* was developed to assist in the preparation for the CELBAN exam.

The CELBAN exam is an English language proficiency exam for internationally educated nurses recognized by Canadian nursing regulators. The exam assesses four areas:

- Speaking
- Listening
- Writing
- Reading

The speaking test takes place separately with two trained assessors. The listening, writing, and reading tests take place in a group setting. This guide will help you to successfully complete the test for the four English language skill areas.

The following chapters cover each of the four skill areas. They include an overview of the format of the test, the criteria used in rating (if available), descriptions of the tasks you need to complete during the test, strategies to successfully complete the tasks, and sample exercises. Information from the CELBAN centre website (www.celbancentre.ca) is included where appropriate.

We wish you all the best as you study and prepare for the exam.

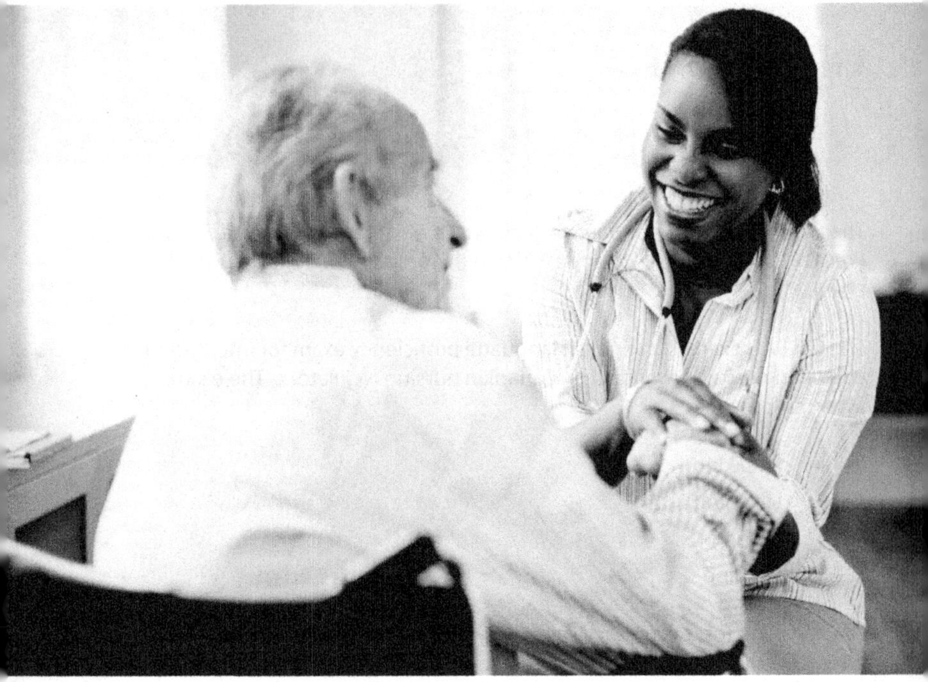

CHAPTER TWO
SPEAKING

Overview

The speaking test is conducted by two speaking assessors. You will engage with them in four types of interactions:

- Introductory questions
- Role plays with nursing scenarios, where you will ask questions to obtain information, give instructions, and offer explanations
- Discussion questions
- Conclusion

It is important to note that only your language proficiency will be assessed, not your medical knowledge. Use accurate nursing-related vocabulary, but don't be concerned with possible mistakes in medical information.

The *Test Information Manual* states that during the speaking test you will "answer questions to demonstrate ability to narrate, describe, summarize, synthesize, state and support opinion, and advise."[1] These are defined as follows:

- To narrate is to tell a story.
- To describe is to say what something or someone is like.
- To summarize is to tell something in fewer words.
- To synthesize is to combine different things (ideas, concepts, treatments, etc.) into one.
- To state is to express something formally in speech or writing.
- To support an opinion is to substantiate or reinforce your position.
- To advise is to recommend or suggest.

The speaking test lasts 20-30 minutes.

[1]http://www.celbancentre.ca/prepare/test-information-manual.aspx (p. 1).

Rating Criteria

The *Test Information Manual* lists the criteria to rate your speaking. These criteria are briefly explained below:

- Communication: Expressing your ideas and opinions clearly so that others can follow.
- Intelligibility: Pronouncing words correctly and using the right stress and intonation.
- Grammar: Ordering and inflecting of words in a sentence correctly.
- Vocabulary: Using appropriate and accurate words to describe ideas or concepts.
- Fluency: Maintaining an even tempo and the avoiding unnecessary pauses.
- Organization and cohesion: Stating the main idea, supporting main points with reasoning or evidence, introducing and concluding, and using words to effectively transition from one point to the next.
- Initiative: Taking initiative for an interaction with confidence.
- Strategies: Ways to communicate effectively.

Introductory Questions

This part of the test you talk for about five minutes in response to a question about yourself. You should:

- Introduce yourself (if you have not already done so).
- Ask for clarity if you are unsure of the question.
- Give an introduction concerning what you are going to talk about.
- Describe your main points in a logical sequence (such as a chronological order of events).
- Conclude with a summary of your answer to the question.

Role Plays

Role plays are like acting in a play. During role plays, one of the assessors will take on the role of a patient or a nurse, and you will assume the role of a nurse (interacting with another nurse or a patient).

For role play exercises, you should:

- Review your scenario script. For example, the script might begin with a patient visit to the hospital or medical clinic.
- Introduce yourself to the patient or nurse. For example: "Hello, my name is … and I will be your nurse today."
- Ask questions or give information according to the script. For example, if the script is about a hospital visit, you will need to ask the reason for the visit (even it is already stated in the script). Questions also need to be asked if the script requires you to complete a patient medical assessment.
- Close the conversation. The conversation should be closed by asking if there are any questions and thanking the nurse or patient for cooperating with you.

The following communication strategies are identified in the *Test Information Manual* for a successful interaction:

- Establish rapport and engage the role player.
- Use appropriate tone, level of formality, and vocabulary for the situation.
- Ask for clarification (ask further questions) to make sure you understand.
- Explain the reasons for your questions and instructions.
- Support any suggestions or directions with a rationale.
- Don't be afraid to correct yourself.
- Be empathetic, but firm.
- Acknowledge the person to whom you are speaking.

Discussion Questions

During this segment of the speaking test, questions will be asked about concepts, ideas, and opinions.

Examples of questions asking your opinion are:

- "Should smoking be allowed in public places?", or
- "Do you agree with the law prohibiting drinking and driving?"

The following format is recommended:

- Repeat or rephrase the question for clarity.
- State your opinion in one sentence. For example, "Yes I think smoking should be allowed in public places."
- Give at least three reasons to support your view and provide examples or evidence. You can also talk about a personal experience.
- Give a conclusion to your opinion. Let the examiner know you have finished by giving a summary or highlighting your main point. For example, "In conclusion, the reasons are why I do not agree..."

Tips for Speaking

For the speaking test, you will be asking questions to gather information. Therefore, it is important to be able to formulate the right kind of question to obtain the information you need. As outlined in the CELBAN Centre tip sheet *Speaking – Asking Questions*,[2] there are generally two types of questions: questions that require only a *yes* or *no* as a response and questions that start with an interrogative word - also known as an WH word. WH words include the "five Ws" *who, what, where, why* and *when* as well as the word *how.*

Here are some examples:

Yes or no questions:

- Are you a smoker?
- Do you drive a vehicle?

WH questions:

- Who should we contact in the case of emergency?
- What is your telephone number?
- Where do you live?
- Why did you come in to the hospital today?
- When did you begin to feel pain?
- How will you be traveling back home?

WH questions are necessary to obtain specific information.

Questions can also be indirect. As stated in the tip sheet, indirect questions are more formal and used to ask sensitive questions. For example, by asking the question, "Do you mind if I ask about your diet?" you are leading up to more direct questions.

It is also common to abbreviate questions if similar questions follow on the same topic and you have the right intonation in your voice. For example: How many children do you have? How many boys? Girls? Any grandchildren?

---

[2]The tip sheets are found at the following link: http://www.celbancentre.ca/prepare/CELBAN-tip-sheets.aspx.

Exercises

Introductory Questions

1. Your Personal Story

Choose one of the following questions to introduce yourself and tell a personal story:

- What is the most frustrating thing about becoming employed as a nurse in Canada?
- Describe the way Edmonton is different from the city or town you grew up in?
- Explain the number one reason you chose to live in Edmonton.

Remember to restate or rephrase the question for clarity if necessary. For example: "Do you mean, what is frustrating with respect to my profession as a nurse?"

Start with an introduction.

Use examples or illustrations. For example: "I must pass the English Language exam as the first step towards becoming a nurse in Canada. That may present a challenge for me because learning a new language is like learning to play a musical instrument..."

End with a conclusion. For example: "It will not be easy, but once I have completed all the steps, then I will enjoy being employed as a nurse in Canada."

Role Play

2. Patient with Chest Pain

You are the nurse working in the emergency department at VPAE hospital. A 70-year-old gentleman walks into the emergency unit with his wife. He tells you that he is experiencing chest pain after shoveling his driveway. He has been clearing snow off his driveway for 30 minutes and then the pain started. You need to assess his condition.

Use the Medical Assessment Form, found at the end of this chapter, to guide your questions and record the patient's responses. Use point form, complete sentences are not required.

One question asks for the current level of pain. Pain must be measured objectively on a scale from one to ten. The question is often phrased as follows: "On a scale of one to ten, with ten being the most unbearable pain, how bad are you feeling?"

3. At the Pharmacist

Your child has been ill for several days with a cough, a fever and a runny nose. You decide that your home remedies are not working, so you go to the pharmacist to ask for help. You want to know whether you should buy medication over the counter or to take your child to your family doctor. You ask the pharmacist for help in making this decision.

Begin this role play by introducing yourself and explaining your situation to the pharmacist. You have 10 minutes. Hint: Give the pharmacist a brief description of your home remedies.

4. Discharge Information

You are the nurse working on Unit 18, the medical unit at VPAE Hospital. Your patient, Ms. O'Neil, is on the medical unit recovering from a heart attack. She will be discharged today.

You are to give diet and medical instructions before she is discharged. This includes the following:

- Eat a heart-healthy diet as instructed by the dietitian.
- Consult your family doctor about when you can begin your exercise program.
- Take your blood pressure medication daily.
- Decrease your alcohol and smoking intake.
- Book a follow up appointment as directed.
- Call for medical help if you have an emergency.

In giving discharge information you are teaching the patient. Usually, this information will be given to you in the script. Take a few moments to read it yourself and become familiar with it so that you can present it to the patient in a conversational style.

Discussion Questions

5. Healthy Eating

Give your opinion on the following: Do you think schools should teach children about healthy eating? Or is this the parents' responsibility?

If necessary, clarify the question by restating or rephrasing. Then begin by stating your opinion on the question. Proceed with main points supported by arguments, examples or illustrations. Summarize your opinion in a concluding statement. You have 20 minutes.

6. Flu Shots

Give your opinion on the following: Should nurses be required by law to take flu shots?

As in the exercise above, state your opinion. Follow with your main points and supporting arguments, examples or illustrations. Conclude by restating your opinion. You have a total of 20 minutes.

Medical Assessment Form

Patient Information

Name:

Age:

Gender: ☐ Male ☐ Female

Reason for Visit

Family Information

Age of Father: Health Status:

Age of Mother: Health Status:

Symptoms Experienced

Additional Health Information

Appetite: Weight Change: Allergies:

Medication Taken

Type: Time/Amount:

Current Level of Pain:

Patient Lifestyle Choices

Drug/Alcohol/Caffeine intake:

Diet:

Smoking:

Exercise:

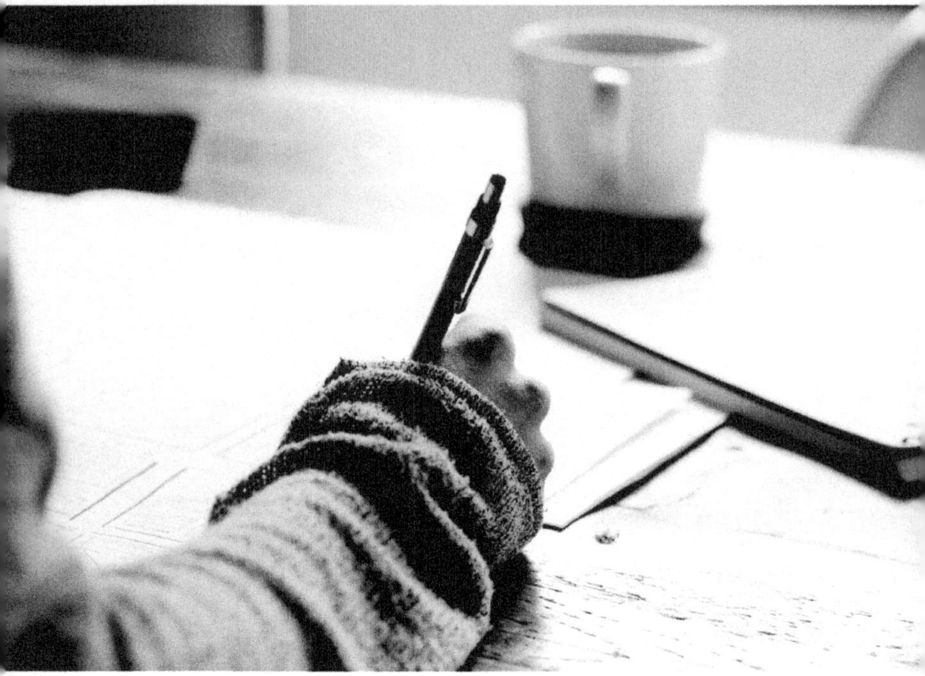

CHAPTER THREE
WRITING

Overview

The writing test includes two tasks; both require you to write complete sentences in paragraph form. Task A is a descriptive writing task. Task B requires you to express and support an opinion.

This segment of the exam takes 45 minutes to complete.

Rating Criteria

The *Test Information Manual* lists the criteria used to rate your writing. These criteria are briefly explained below:

- Task purpose - whether your written response meets the task requirement.
- Content and organization - whether your writing is structured in a manner that connects ideas together so that it is easy for the reader to understand.
- Grammatical structures - whether you use a variety of sentence structures and follow rules of grammar.
- Vocabulary, word forms and usage - whether the words you use demonstrate variety of general and health-related vocabulary, are the right words based on their meaning, and written in correct grammatical form.
- Overall impression and fluency - whether your writing flows well, making it easy for the reader to follow and understand.

Tips for Writing

The CELBAN Centre provides two tip sheets for the writing test: one concerning the organization of your writing and the other on the use of parallel structure.

Advice on the organization of your writing focuses on the completeness and logical progression of ideas in your writing. Suggestions include the following (with examples provided):

- Sequence/order. "Let me outline what happened to the patient. First, he was admitted to the hospital. Second..."
- Reinforcement/similarity. "The pain was excruciating, like the pain of child birth."
- Alternative/contract. "There is a history of heart disease in her family; however, she is currently living an active, healthy lifestyle."
- Example. "He has struggles with anger management. For example, the other day in school he threw a pencil at another student that told him his answer was wrong."
- Result/consequence. "His diet consists mostly of fast foods and processed foods. As a result, he is at risk of diabetes."
- Summary/conclusion. "To summarize, because of consistent exercise and changes to her diet, her heart rate and blood pressure has come down."

Advice on the use of parallel structure refers to a similar grammatical structure at various levels in your writing. Within a sentence, words serving the same grammatical function should be parallel. For example, the nurse was calm, cool and collected.

Parallelism also applies to phrases and clauses. For example: "She was lying in the bed, reading a book and sipping her drink." Bulleted lists should also have a parallel grammatical structure.

Exercises

1. Patient with Sore Throat

You are working in the Emergency Department of the hospital. You have just completed an interview with Ms. Smith who reported having a sore throat for the past three days. Use the words and phrases below to write a descriptive paragraph about Ms. Smith's health. Use complete sentences.

- Pain
- Fever
- Headache
- Nausea
- Vomiting
- Tylenol two tablets
- Loss of appetite

2. Article on Wounds

Write two paragraphs (in about 100 words) describing what the following article is about. Use complete sentences.

WOUNDS[3]

By Amy H. Kaji, MD, PhD, Associate Professor, Department of Emergency Medicine, Harbor-UCLA Medical Center
Cuts or tears in tissue (lacerations), scrapes (abrasions), and puncture wounds can be caused by bites or by other mechanisms. Wounds that are not caused by bites and are clean and relatively small usually heal rapidly without any problems. However, some wounds can cause extensive blood loss.

In some wounds, deeper structures, such as nerves, tendons, or blood vessels, are also injured. Other wounds can become infected. A piece of foreign material (such as a splinter, glass, or a clothing fragment) can also remain hidden inside a wound, causing later problems such as infection.

Shallow cuts to most areas of the skin rarely bleed much and often stop bleeding on their own. Cuts to the hand and scalp as well as cuts to arteries and larger veins often bleed vigorously.

Infection can develop when a wound is contaminated with dirt and bacteria. Although any wound can become infected, infection is particularly likely in deep scrapes, which grind dirt into the skin, and in puncture wounds

[3]https://www.merckmanuals.com/home/injuries-and-poisoning/first-aid/wounds

(particularly those resulting from animal bites or human bites), which introduce contamination deep under the skin. Also, wounds that contain foreign material frequently become infected. The longer a wound remains contaminated, the more likely it is that infection will develop.

Wounds can be painful at first, but usually the pain lessens after the first day. If a cut affects a nerve or tendon, the person may be unable to move the body part fully. Some nerve injuries cause weakness or paralysis, loss of sensation, or numbness. If foreign material remains inside a puncture wound, the part of the wound near the material is usually painful when touched.

Pain that worsens a day or more after the injury is often the first sign of infection. Later, an infected wound becomes red and swollen and may ooze pus. A fever may also develop.

Necrotizing skin infections are rapidly progressing infections that threaten life and limb that can occur even after a very minor skin wound.

3. Head Injury

You are the nurse working in the emergency department at the Children's Hospital called Teddy Bear. At 22:15 Robert, a four-year-old boy, was brought in by his mother. She told you her son had been hit on the head after supper while playing with his older brother in the backyard.

Robert had these symptoms:

- Fever
- Lethargic
- Confusion
- Headache
- Sensitivity to light
- Stiff neck

Using complete sentences, write two paragraphs (approximately 100 words) describing Robert's condition as presented. Include the symptoms listed above. Report your actions as interventions as the nurse on duty.

4. Patient with Chest Pain

A 70-year-old man walks into the Emergency Unit on your day shift. He complained of chest pain after clearing his drive way of snow. His wife drove him to emergency. Write a descriptive report using the following words and phrases:

- Non-smoker
- Family history of high cholesterol and heart attack
- Aspirin medication prescribed once per day
- Nitroglycerin given in emergency
- Consumption of alcohol

5. Patient on the Floor

You are the night nurse on duty 2300 hours to 0700 hours. Your responsibilities include supervision of staff, patient care supervision and management of sick calls for the replacement of day shift. Patient supervision on night shift is done every two hours by staff. On your third patient night check, you found Ms. Brown sitting quietly on the floor beside her bed at 0300 hours.

Write one to two paragraphs about this incident. Use complete sentences and include the following in your report:

- The scenario (note that there were no witnesses present).
- The setting and Location: the time, place and date (use today's date).
- The patient's condition.
- The following vital signs: Blood Pressure = 120/80, Respiration = 16, Pulse = 80, Physical Status = Responsive

6. Smoking

In paragraph form, state and support your opining on the following question: Should smoking be allowed in public places? Use complete sentences.

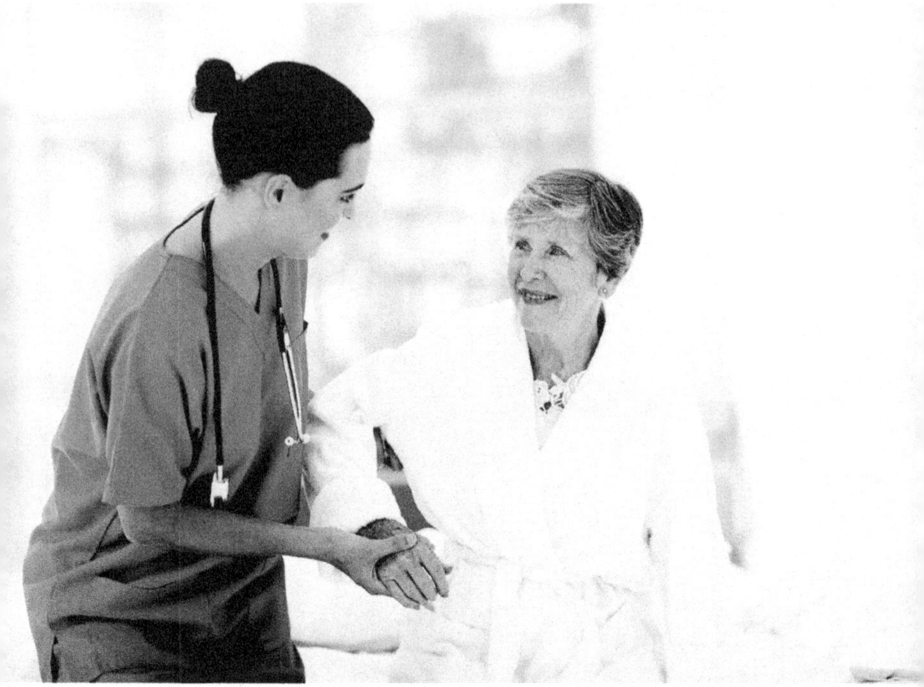

CHAPTER FOUR
LISTENING

Overview

During the listening test a series of four audio and five video clips will be played, which portray interactions between nurses and patients, family members, and other professionals. The four audio clips include phone calls and shift reports.

You will be given a test booklet to record answers to multiple choice questions. Each audio or video clip is only played once. However, you will be given time to review the questions in advance.

The listening test takes 45 minutes to complete.

Tips for Listening

The *Test Information Manual* provides the following advice:

- Pre-read questions before viewing or listening to the scenarios.
- Mark answers in your test booklet as soon as you hear the information needed. View the video, read the questions, and select your answers at the same time.
- Use the dedicated time at the end of each scenario to check your answers. Do not use the time allotted for pre-reading to look at the next questions for the next task.

Remember listening requires concentration. Rather than watching the video as you would a movie, focus on the listening to the audio or video and answering the questions as you are listening.

Exercises

The exercises below are shift reports to give you practice listening and answer multiple-choice questions. This is the essential skill required for video and audio listening tasks in the exam.

The audio clips are available on-line through the VPAE website at the following link:

http://vocationalpathways.ca/guide.html

Choose the best answer from multiple choice options. Circle your response and only change your answer if you are sure your first choice is incorrect.

Note: the audio recordings are transcribed below for your reference, but focus on the audio clip, not the written text.

1. Night Shift Report

This is the night shift report for Unit 11C by Madeline Weary.

At 0300 hours when the night shift nurse was doing the hourly patient night check, Mrs. Brown in Room 12A, Bed 2 was found on the floor in her room in a sitting position, between her bed and the night table. There were no bruises noted. Vital signs taken and all within normal limits. Patient stated she was reaching for a drink of water on the night table, when she slipped out of bed. No witnesses present.

She was assisted back to bed with instructions to use the call bell to ask for help. She slept the remaining of the night shift and voiced no concerns. Dr. Peter Dion and patient's daughter notified of incident. Doctor's orders are to continue to observe patient's behaviour and monitor vital signs for any changes.

End of night shift report

Madeline Weary, LPN

Questions

1. What is the patient's name?
   a. Weary
   b. Madeline
   c. Brown

2. What hospital Unit are they in?
   a. 12A
   b. 11C
   c. 11D

3. What time did the incident occur?
   a. 1300
   b. 0003
   c. 0300

4. What room is the patient in?
   a. 12A
   b. 11C
   c. 2B

5. What is doctor's name?
   a. Peter Dean
   b. Peter Dion
   c. Peter One

6. Where was the patient found when the incident occurred?
   a. Beside night table
   b. Floor
   c. Bed

7. What is the nurse's name?
   a. Wear
   b. Madeline
   c. Brown

8. What bed is the patient in?
   a. Too
   b. To
   c. Two

2. Evening Shift Report

Evening shift report by Felisha-Ann Smith.

This is the evening shift report for the Emergency Unit EMR 3.

At 2215 hours Robert Miller, a 4-year-old boy, was brought into the EMR 3 Unit carried by his mother, Mrs. Mary Miller. She stated that Robert had been hit on the head after supper, while playing with his older brother in the back yard of the family home. She stated she had applied a cold pack to Robert's head as she suspected swelling. No swelling or bleeding noted upon patient's arrival. Patient presented with the following symptoms: fever of 38.2° C, complaining of headache, and pain in the back of the neck and head. States pain is 7 out of 10. Lethargic and unable to stand by himself.

Dr. Charles Wesley, the doctor on call, was notified and he ordered the following: children's Tylenol for fever and pain—10 ml to be given right away, and every 4 hours as needed. CT Scan Stat, and to monitor vital signs every 4 hours. To notify him immediately if Robert's condition deteriorates. Robert's first dose of Tylenol was given at 2230, and his temperature was 38.0° C. Robert is in Room 2, Bed 4 with his mother sitting beside him. She wants to spend the night at the hospital in the room with him. I think you will enjoy being their nurse tonight.

Good luck. Bye.

End of the evening shift report.

Felisha-Ann Smith

Questions

1. What is the patient's name?
   a. Roberta Miller
   b. Robert Mill
   c. Robert Miller

2. What is the age of the patient?
   a. Infant
   b. Toddler
   c. Four

3. Where is the patient injured?
   a. Neck and head
   b. Neck
   c. Head only

4. What was the patient's initial temperature?
   a. 38.0° C
   b. 38.2° C
   c. 38.1° C

5. What does it mean that the patient is lethargic?
   a. Patient is sleeping
   b. Patient is drowsy
   c. Patient is in a bad mood

6. What is the doctor's name?
   a. Charles Weslin
   b. Charles Wesley
   c. Charles Wesler

7. What is the doctor's status?
   a. Family Doctor
   b. Doctor on Call
   c. Hospital Doctor

8. What room is the patient in?
   a. 4
   b. 2
   c. 1

9. What bed is the patient in?
   a. 2
   b. 4
   c. 3

10. What is the nurse's name?
   a. Ann
   b. Felisha-Ann
   c. Felisha

11. What is the patient's pain level?
   a. 8 out of 10
   b. 7 out of 10
   c. 6 out of 10

12. When did the patient arrive?
   a. 2230
   b. 2215
   c. 2200

13. What is the name of the patient's mother?
   a. Mary Milley
   b. Marlene Miller
   c. Mary Miller

14. What time was medication delivered to the patient?
   a. 2215
   b. 2200
   c. 2230

3. Afternoon Shift Report

Afternoon shift report by Cassandra Leeman

This is the afternoon shift report for the Emergency Unit EMR 1.

At 1526 hours Jennifer Talbot aged 19 was brought into the EMR 1 Unit by ambulance with EMR attendants and her mother Mrs. Elizabeth Talbot. According to Mrs. Talbot, Jennifer was found unconscious in her bedroom at home around 1500 hours. Jennifer had a kidney dialysis two weeks ago performed by Dr. Manny Patai. She was born with kidney disease and is cared for by her mother. Jennifer was conscious when she arrived at the hospital and has been placed in Room 11, Bed 3 in Ward 6H. Dr. Manny Patai was informed of her hospitalization and will be assessing her need for another dialysis tomorrow, Tuesday, August 4th.

In the meantime, the attending Emergency physician Dr. Ronda Wilker has advised rest for Jennifer, and no medical treatments beyond her regular medicine. Jennifer is having difficulty seeing clearly and is seeing double. She is also short of breath and finding it hard to concentrate and answer questions about her condition. Once she was placed in her room her mother left the hospital and is planning to return this evening around 2000 hours.

End of the afternoon shift report.

Cassandra Leeman, RN

Questions

1. What is the patient's name?
   a. Mrs. Elizabeth Talbot
   b. Jennifer Talbot
   c. Cassandra Leeman

2. What hospital Unit is she in?
   a. Unit 1
   b. Ward 6H
   c. Room 11

3. What was the reason for patient's arrival at the hospital?
   a. Kidney failure
   b. Kidney dialysis
   c. Found unconscious in her room

4. What is the name of the attending physician?
    a. Dr. Manny Patai
    b. Dr. Ronda Wilker
    c. Dr. Elizabeth Talbot

5. How did the patient arrive at the hospital?
    a. She was brought in by her mother.
    b. She came in by herself.
    c. She arrived in ambulance.

6. What is the nurse's name?
    a. Cassandra Leeman
    b. Jennifer Talbot
    c. Manny Patai

7. What chronic condition does the patient have?
    a. Vision trouble and difficulty breathing and speaking.
    b. Kidney disease.
    c. She is unconscious.

8. What time did the patient arrive at the hospital?
    a. 2000 hours
    b. 1500 hours
    c. 1526 hours
    d.

9. What did the attending physician advise for the patient?
    a. Rest and recuperation.
    b. Kidney dialysis.
    c. Vision treatment.

4. Morning Shift Report

Morning shift report by Claude Fort.

This is the morning shift report for Unit 5B

At 0936 hours Gordon Erickson age 68, who has cancer of the esophagus and is due for surgery in three days, pressed the call bell. I went to check on him immediately and he informed me that he had just spent the last five minutes vomiting in the bed pan at the side of his bed. I called in some health care aides to replace the bed pan and clean the side of his bed and the floor. Gordon said he no longer felt nauseous but was very dizzy. I rinsed out his mouth and gave him a gravel and some water. His appetite has been inconsistent and he has not eaten since breakfast at 0700.

His pathologist is Dr. Mary Lewis, and his surgeon will be Dr. Phil Clarke. Drs. Lewis and Clarke have indicated that it would be ideal if he could consume at least 500 calories a day to keep his strength up for surgical recovery. Gordon has been sleeping most of the day but encouraged him to eat supper when he wakes up.

End of morning shift report.

Claude Fort, LPN

Questions

1. What is the patient's name?
    a. Lewis Clarke
    b. Claude Fort
    c. Gordon Erickson

2. What is the name of the patient's surgeon?
    a. Dr. Phil Clarke
    b. Dr. Claude Fort
    c. Dr. Mary Lewis

3. What time did the incident occur?
   a. 0900 hours
   b. 0936 hours
   c. 0930 hours

4. What is the name of the patient's pathologist?
   a. Dr. Mary Lewis
   b. Dr. Gordon Erickson
   c. Dr. Phil Clarke

5. What is patient's current condition as of the end of the report?
   a. He is nauseous and dizzy.
   b. He is sleeping and has for most of the day.
   c. He is hungry.

6. What is the nurse's name?
   a. Claude Fort
   b. Mary Lewis
   c. Phil Clarke

7. What is the nurse's recommendation in the report?
   a. Let the patient sleep as much as possible.
   b. Have the patient's pathologist check in on him.
   c. Encourage the patient to eat when he wakes up.

8. What time did the patient arrive at the hospital?
   a. 0936 hours
   b. 0700 hours
   c. He was hospitalized previous to this report.

9. What is the doctor's recommendation for the patient mentioned in the report?
   a. To eat at least 500 calories a day.
   b. Rest and recuperation.
   c. Surgical treatment.

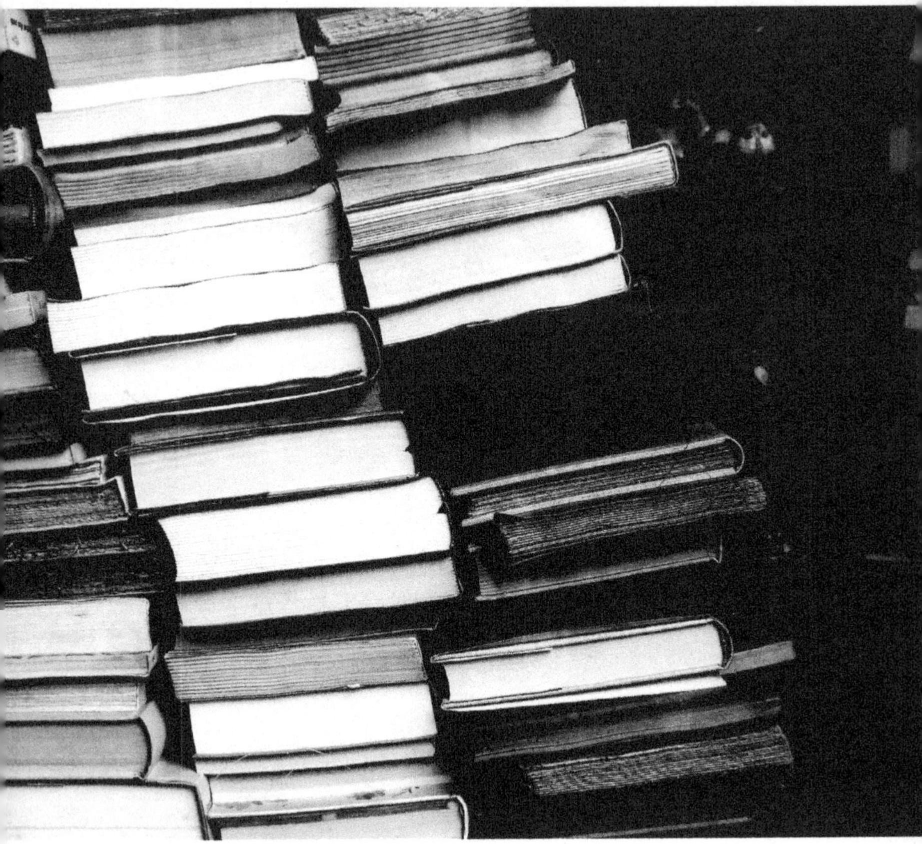

CHAPTER FIVE
READING

Overview

The reading test involves a series of health-related text passages, each followed by multiple choice questions. Texts include charts, patient notes, manuals, and short articles related to healthcare. You will also complete a fill-in-the-blanks exercise with multiple choice options.

In some of the reading tasks you need to skim and scan the text to find the answers to the questions. In other reading tasks you need to read the entire text to answer the questions.

The reading test takes 60 minutes to complete.

Tips for Reading

It is likely that you will come across new words as you take the reading test. The CELBAN Center provides a tip sheet that provides some advice on how to determine the meaning of a word from its context. Strategies include looking for clues to the meaning of a word by focusing on the phrases surrounding the word, identify the grammatical function of the word (whether it is a noun, verb, adjective or adverb), look for synonyms within the sentence, and look for logical clues.

For example, if a patient is described as "sanguine, expecting to recover quickly" you could infer from the words that follow sanguine that it means optimistic. Or if someone is described as "dispassionate, unlike [another person] who is empathetic" you can understand the word dispassionate from the opposite word empathetic.

Exercises

Skimming and Scanning

1. Gastroscopy Preparation

You are given five minutes to review the patient gastroscopy preparation instructions below:

Name: Ms. Lydia Awassa
Date of appointment: Monday, August 7, 2011
Time of arrival: 12:30 pm
Procedure start time: 1:45pm
Patient must report to: Joan Clarkson at the patient registration desk located in the hospital lobby front entrance.
Day before instructions: After 6pm refrain from eating solid foods; the following may be consumed as clear fluids up to midnight: water, Jello, fruit juice, hot beverages without milk or cream.
Day of test instructions: Please do not eat or drink.
Transportation home instructions: Arrange to have assistance to take you home after the procedure, as the procedure requires sedation and you will not be able to drive.

Answer the following questions:

- What is the name of the patient?
- What is the patient procedural time?
- What is the name of the person the patient must report to?
- Where is the patient registration desk located?
- What are the patient instructions for the day of the test?
- Why is a transportation agreement necessary?
- What is the appointment date?

2. Outpatient Registration Information

You are given five minutes to review the outpatient registration information below:

Chart No.: 765-345
Patient First name: Theresa- Ann
Patient Last name: Riley
Middle initial: J
Address: Mountain View Crescent
City: Spring View
Postal Code: T56 2PS
Home Phone: 780-123-7891
Work phone: 780-123-112 Extension: 00
Cellular Phone: 999-666-1112
Date of Birth: 1955/11/30
Emergency Contact: Spouse
Name: Harold Riley
Telephone: Same as home number

Answer the following questions:

- What is the name of the patient?
- What is the patients chart number?
- What is the telephone number for the patient's spouse?
- What is the name of the city the patient resides in?
- What is the patients home address?
- What year was the patient born?

Vocabulary and Comprehension

3. Diet and Nutrition

Read the article below, and then answer the multiple choice questions. Choose the best answer by circling your choice. You have 15 minutes.

Types of Nutrients

There are six general types of nutrients. Three of these nutrients supply the body with energy, the other three nutrients regulate body processes.

Nutrients Used for Energy

1. Carbohydrates
2. Protein
3. Fats (Lipids)

Nutrients used for energy

1. Vitamins
2. Minerals
3. Water

Water

Water is provided in the diet in the form of beverages; coffee, tea, ice cream, soups, milk, pop and water. Water is also found in many fruits and vegetables. Water provides no calories or nutrition, but water is essential to life. We can only live for three to seven days without water

Function of water

1. Transportation: Nutrients found in foods are dissolved in water and other fluids found in the body. Water moves these nutrients in and out of the body cells.
2. Excretion: Water removes waste products such as urine and feces from the body
3. Lubricant: Water keeps the internal organs moist, prevents friction between moving body parts, and keeps the joints moving freely.

Canada Food Guide

For optimum nutritional health our body requires a diet that provides a balanced amount of essential nutrients found in the foods we eat. Two tools are available to help us achieve this goal. The Canada Food Guide, and the nutritional labels on foods. Canada's Food Guide is a nutritional food plan to be used to assist us to meet the nutritional needs of the body. It involves following a daily food plan that is based on four food groups. A specific number of servings of food from each of the four food groups are recommended on a daily basis. Canada's Food Guide is inclusive of food choices that represent different cultural groups represented in Canada

Food Labels

The second tool available to assist with planning a balanced diet is the nutritional labels that are found on most foods. The labels provide nutritional information of the food's nutritional value, approximate serving size, and any health-related claims. By reading the food label helps us to make better food choices for the day in meeting our nutritional goals.

Types of Diets

There are three types of basic diets.

1. The Regular Diet: The regular diet contains the four basic food groups, supplying the client with an adequate amount of nutrients required to meet the nutritional needs of the body. Usually there are no restrictions found in this diet except for the client's food preferences, which may include cultural preferences, likes and dislikes.
2. Modified and special diets: Modified diets are similar to the regular diet, in that the food choices are based upon the four food groups in the Canada Food Guide. However, the texture of the food is changed to meet the individual client's digestive needs of swallowing and chewing. Foods may be chopped, minced (ground) or pureed (blended) soft diets (modified diet) are foods that are not highly seasoned, fried, or high in fiber; as the diet has been changed to remove foods that are hard to chew or swallow. Clear liquid diets (special diet) do not contain enough nutrients to maintain optimum health for a long time. A client may only be on this diet for a short period of time. Clear liquids are substances that can be poured at room temperature. Examples of foods considered clear fluids are; water, gelatin, fat free broth, or bouillon, popsicles, clear juices, tea or coffee without cream. A client who is nauseous, or vomiting, or who has just returned from surgery may be put on this diet by their doctor. Full liquid diets (special diets) are clear liquid diets with the additional foods that can be poured at room temperature. Examples of foods that can be poured at room temperature are; milk, frozen yogurt, custard, and eggnog. A client may be on this type of diet plan for three or more days with a high protein liquid dietary supplement.
3. Therapeutic diets: A therapeutic diet meets a special nutritional need for a client's specific illness. A particular component part of the diet is designed

to address the client's condition or illness. Some examples of therapeutic diets are; Sodium Restricted diet, Low Cholesterol diet, and the diabetic diet. Sodium Restricted diets used for the treatment of heart disease, hypertension, and kidney disease. A client on a sodium restricted diet may be allowed to have small amounts of salt or none at all. Low Cholesterol diet is for clients who are unable to digest or use fat; a low-fat diet may be ordered. Foods are chosen that are lower in animal fat and prepared in ways that do not add additional fats. Butter, margarine, and shortening are avoided, and foods such as fruits, vegetables, wholegrains, and skim milk are encouraged in the meal plan. The Diabetic diet regulates the amount of fat, carbohydrates, and protein a client needs. The diet plan is different for each client as this is based upon the nutritional requirement and energy level of the client and this is reflected in the clients care plan.

Nutritional supplements

Some clients will require nutritional supplements that are offered either before or after meals. These nutritional supplements are usually in the form of flavoured shakes and drinks. Quite often diabetic clients are required to have nutritional supplements between meals to keep their blood sugar levels stable.[4]

[4]Adapted from Pamela Carter and Marilyn McGreer (ed), *Lippincott's Textbook for Personal Support Workers* (Lippincott: Philadelphia, 2011), pp. 372-380.

Multiple Choice Questions (Choose the Best Answer)

1. Carbohydrate nutrition is best described as:
   a. The intake of food in the body
   b. The process of how food intake is used in the body
   c. Chemical substances and their use in the body
   d. Nutrients used as energy for the body

2. Water is vital to our body because:
   a. All cells of the body contain water
   b. Foods contain water that our body can use
   c. Water helps us lose weight
   d. Water assists in important functions of the body

3. The main purpose of different types of diets is to:
   a. Give the client more options to choose
   b. Assist the client in their weight management program
   c. Assist the client with their chewing and swallowing difficulties
   d. Assist the client in meeting the nutritional demands of their body

4. Canada Food Guide is inclusive of food choices:
   a. To represent Canada's ethnic diversity of people
   b. To emphasize the importance of pleasing everyone
   c. To identify the importance of food choices
   d. Only a and c are correct

5. The article is best described as:
   a. Food and nutrition
   b. The importance of eating well
   c. Canada Food Guide and labels
   d. None of the above

Fill in the Blanks

4. New Perspective on Smoking

Read the paragraph below and choose the correct word for each blank by circling the answer below the paragraph. You are given five minutes to complete this assignment.

Smoking __1__ taken on a new image. At one time smoking __2___ considered to have __3__glamourous image everyone wanted to adopt. Research of the twenty first century __4__destroyed that movie star image by showing the devastating effects of smoking ___5___ to the body. The medical research shows that second hand smoke ___6___ is also directly related to __7___respiratory diseases and problems; such __8___ lung cancer. The government __9__ taken steps to protect the public through legislation. Smoking bans ___10___ in place in most jurisdictions. It is not uncommon ___11___ see __12____ non- smoking sign in__13__ restaurant __14___ washroom facility. These facilities __15___ considered to be public places __16__ __17___ spaces __18___ all age groups of people use and enjoy.

1. a. have b. has c. had

2. a. were b. was c. where

3. a. an b. a c. and

4. a. have b. has c. had

5. a. is b. are c. a

6. a. is b. a c. are

7. a. too b. to c. two

8. a. had b. as c. has

9. a. has b. have c. had

10. a. is b. are c. was

11. a. to b. too c. two

12. a. an b. a c. and

13. a. a b. an c. and

14. a. and b. an c. a

15. a. are b. is c. a;

16. a. where b. were c. wear

17. a. of b. off c. for

18. a) are b) is c) of

Made in the USA
Monee, IL
04 November 2026

67384273R00030